Sleep disordered breathing

A parent's guide

Dr David McIntosh

MBBS
FRACS
PhD

Pediatric ENT Surgeon

For Sophie and Adam- my reason for being

Please consult with a qualified healthcare professional regarding any specific medical concerns or questions you may have

Contents

1. Introduction

My name is David. I am a pediatric ear nose and throat surgeon in Queensland, Australia. I have been helping children and their families navigate their way through a diagnosis for sleep disordered breathing for over 30 years now. During that time my understanding and awareness of the condition, its management, and its consequences if left untreated, have grown substantially. Now I want to share the benefits of these 30 years of experience with you. I will do so being mindful that I am not your child's doctor, so please make sure you use the information here as a guide rather than as an absolute recommendation.

In introducing myself to you, I just want to say that I have thoroughly enjoyed writing this book. Feedback from friends and colleagues is that it is going to be a very helpful resource for families throughout the world. They were too polite to say it, but at times I will admit I am a bit opinionated and may even sound a bit patronizing. I have been doing this for a long time and I just know too much to not want to share my knowledge, and if at times you find it a bit high and mighty of me, well just know that it is all written in the best of faith of wanting you to know what I think is best for you to know to help get you and your child through the diagnosis and management of this condition. So be kind to me and accept my failings for being opinionated at times. Oh, and I can be flippant at times. Just soak it up.

In this book I will explain what sleep disordered breathing is, what causes it, what problems it causes to a child, and how we assess a child for a cause of their sleep disordered breathing to then determine the best pathway to achieve better breathing and sleep. To do this, I want to start off with a story.

Once upon a time, in a small town near one of Australia's iconic beaches, there lived a curious and caring parent named Ashleigh. Ashleigh had noticed that her beloved child, Lilly, had been snoring loudly during the night when they went camping one weekend. She hadn't noticed this before, and decided to watch over Lilly for the next few nights when they got home. She noticed the snoring was happening each night. After doing some online searching, Ashleigh was concerned about Lilly's well-being, and decided to take her to see an Ear, Nose, and Throat (ENT) specialist to get some answers.

So, one sunny morning, after her and Lilly had been for a swim at the beach, they both embarked on their journey to the ENT clinic. As they entered the waiting room, they were greeted by friendly smiles from the staff and a warm and welcoming atmosphere. There were a lot of parents and children waiting to be seen. Ashleigh could feel a sense of comfort and confidence growing within her that she was in the right place.

Soon, it was Lilly's turn to meet the ENT specialist, Dr. David. With a friendly demeanor, Dr. David invited them into the examination room. Ashleigh explained her concerns about Lilly's snoring and how she had done some online research and wondered if it had been affecting her sleep quality and overall well-being, as Lilly had become less of the angel she used to be in the past few months and Ashleigh did not understand why this was the case.

Dr. David listened attentively, nodding understandingly. He explained to Ashleigh that snoring in children can be indicative of a larger issue, such as obstructive sleep apnea or enlarged tonsils or adenoids. He assured Ashleigh that they would conduct a thorough assessment to determine the cause of the snoring and recommend the best course of action.

Dr. David carefully examined Lilly's ears, nose, and throat. He told her he was looking for mermaids, as they had been for a swim that morning. This made Lilly giggle. He also asked about Lilly's sleep patterns, daytime energy levels, and any other symptoms she might have been experiencing related to ger emotions, concentration, and focus. After the examination, Dr. David sat down with Ashleigh and Lilly to share his findings.

"Ashleigh," Dr. David began, "Lilly's snoring is due to enlarged tonsils that I saw when I looked inside her throat. At the back of her nose, the adenoids look to be too large as well. This is probably causing disruptions in her sleep patterns and leading to various symptoms such as daytime sleepiness, mood changes, and difficulty concentrating."

Ashleigh felt a mix of relief and concern. She was relieved that they had finally identified the cause of Lilly's snoring, but concerned about the impact it might have on her daughter's health and well-being.

Dr. David reassured Ashleigh, "The good news is that we can help Lilly. I recommend a tonsillectomy and adenoidectomy to remove her enlarged tonsils and adenoids. It's now the most common type of surgical procedure performed on children in Australia and this is the most common reason we perform it. I know you said she hasn't had tonsillitis, but that is a different problem and a different reason we do the operation. Sometimes, and this is one of those times, we can have the same operation, but for different indications.

Ashleigh listened intently as Dr. David explained the procedure, the recovery process, and the potential benefits it would bring to Lilly's overall health and quality of life. She felt a growing sense of confidence in Dr. David's expertise and knew that this was the right decision for Lilly.

With gratitude, Ashleigh thanked Dr. David for his thorough examination and guidance. She felt a renewed sense of hope and relief, knowing that they were on the path to helping Lilly overcome her snoring and the underlying issues causing it.

In the weeks that followed, Lilly underwent the surgery. Ashleigh supported her every step of the way, providing comfort, love, and encouragement during the recovery process. And ice cream. Lots of ice cream. Lilly's snoring gradually faded away, replaced by peaceful nights and restful sleep.

As time went on, Lilly's overall well-being improved significantly. She felt more energetic during the day, her concentration and school performance improved, and she woke up feeling refreshed and ready to take on new adventures. The whole family rejoiced in Lilly's newfound vitality and happiness.

Ashleigh realized the importance of addressing concerns and seeking help when it came to her child's health. Through the journey of taking Lilly to see the ENT specialist, she learned the power of trust, communication, and advocating for her child's well-being. She also realized that like her, other parents may not even know that snoring in children is a source of concern and decided to make sure her friends and family knew to look out for the warning signs such as mouth breathing, snoring, and waking up tired and cranky and then struggling through the day.

As simple as this narrative is, it is indeed a helpful summation of the journey of many children that are diagnosed with sleep disordered breathing, it is by no means the while story. So, let's go and learn a bit more.

2. Normal breathing

In order to understand a problem, one needs to know what is normal and, in this context, it is breathing and sleep that need to be elaborated upon, so let's start with breathing in this chapter, and we will cover sleep in the next.

For most of us, breathing comes naturally and happens normally. That is thanks to our brain, specifically a part of it known as the respiratory center. It is located towards the back and lower part of the brain. Although the regulation of breathing is a complex process the following is a simplified explanation of how breathing is controlled.

A special part of the brain generates the basic rhythm of breathing. It sends a signal via nerves to the muscles involved in breathing, specifically the diaphragm and muscles between the ribs. This part of the brain responds to messages it gets from certain monitors set up in the brain and throughout the body. The main thing that the brain wants to know about, surprisingly, is not oxygen, but the waste product of our body's metabolism called carbon dioxide. Carbon dioxide levels are very important because when it mixes with water, it can lead to a chemical reaction that forms an acid, and this acid can lead to a change in the pH of the blood and cells in the body. If this happens, then the way the whole-body functions can be disrupted, so it is important to protect against this adverse event from arising.

Breathing is really quite magical. If the carbon dioxide levels go up, then there is a subtle change in the blood pH, just a smidge. But that small change is enough to get the respiratory center's attention and it responds by changing the rate of breathing and increasing it. Every time we breathe out, our body is getting rid of some of this carbon dioxide. So, it is a brilliant system in keeping things in equilibrium.

The bonus of all of this is that breathing also allows us to take in oxygen, the vital ingredient for our cells to work the way they do. Without oxygen we would rapidly die. The advantage of this all happening automatically means we have the luxury of going to sleep, and the brain just keeps ticking over in maintaining our breathing. If we had to consciously think about breathing all the time, we would not survive when we fall asleep. In Greek mythology, such a curse was placed by Ondine upon her unfaithful husband, compelling him to forever stay awake so that he could breathe-talk about torture!

3. Normal sleep

You may be surprised to learn that we did not know much about sleep from a scientific point of view until the past 100 years, and more so the past 50, and even more so the past 25. Rather than being a period of dormancy, where nothing happens, our brain goes through a remarkable sequence of deliberated structured stages that we are still to fully understand. However, as we are keeping this simple, fortunately there is enough we know to do just that.

So, to start off with, sleep is divided in stages depending on the measurements of electrical activity in the brain. The two broad divisions of brain activity fall into Rapid Eye Movement (REM) sleep and Non-Rapid Eye Movement (NREM) sleep. These cycles repeat throughout the night, typically in a pattern of around 90 minutes. Let's go through these in a bit more detail.

REM sleep is characterized by rapid eye movements and increased brain activity resembling wakefulness. This is when most of our dreaming occurs. As we can measure the brain wave patterns and know when a test subject is in a certain stage of sleep, researches have explored the consequences of depriving someone of their REM sleep by waking them up when it was evident on the brain waves. Based on the testing of such subjects, it is now inferred that REM sleep is important for cognitive functions, certain types of memory consolidation, and emotional regulation. So, in other words, poor quality or inadequate quality of REM sleep leads to day time functioning problems in those afflicted by disruption to their REM sleep. Keep this in mind as we progress further in the book and talk about the effects of sleep disordered breathing.

NREM Sleep is not just one type of brain wave pattern but can be divided up into 3 subsections, or stages, known simply as: N1, N2, and N3. N1 (also known as Stage 1) is the stepping stone in time from being awake to falling asleep. It is a light sleep stage, and people can easily be awakened from this stage. N2 (also known as Stage 2) is also light sleep but it is the main stage of light sleep. It also is where we spend most of our time when we are asleep. During this stage, the body enters into a state of relaxation, and we find that the heart rate slows down, and body temperature decreases. Then we have N3 (also known as Stage 3). N3 is also known as deep sleep. It is the deepest and most restorative stage of sleep, essential for physical and mental rejuvenation. It is harder to wake someone during this stage, and as an aside, this is when sleepwalking or bedwetting may occur.

Although there are 4 elements or stages of sleep (REM and the three NREM stages), the flow of the sleep pattern is not as you might predict. Initially we do have N1, followed by N2 and then N3, but then we bounce back to N2, and then land in REM sleep. This is known as the sleep cycle. Interestingly, even though this cycle repeats itself every 90 minutes or so, during each subsequent cycle, there is slightly longer REM stage and shorter N3 (deep sleep stage) each time it cycles through.

In a typical night's sleep, NREM sleep accounts for about 75-80% of total sleep time, and REM sleep accounts for about 20-25% of total sleep time. Regardless of this all happening by itself, there are many things that can happen that can disrupt this sleep pattern, also known as sleep architecture. In due course we will be talking about something called sleep hygiene. For now, just know that it's important to maintain a regular sleep schedule and ensure an adequate amount of sleep each night to support overall health and well-being.

4. Overview of Sleep-Disordered Breathing: obstructive sleep apnea (OSA), upper airways resistance syndrome, snoring, and mouth breathing

Now you might have noticed that those last chapters were pretty brief. That is all about to change. The recommended step from here is just work your way slowly through the rest of the book. As you do so, there may be questions about certain things that come to mind. That is both normal and good. Write them down, and put them to the side temporarily-towards the end of this book there is a whole section on frequently asked questions, so hopefully you will find answers to what you were wondering about. Oh, and of course you can just jump forwards and have a look sooner than later if your curiosity is really getting to you. OK, sleep disordered breathing, the reason we came here in the first place.

Sleep disordered breathing is an overarching term that describes a spectrum of severity of airway obstruction. Now whilst there may be a spectrum of the severity, none of it is good- think of it like comparing being hit by a car versus by a truck. The comparison is somewhat pointless as to adverse outcomes when the consequences range from bad to really bad.

Pediatric sleep-disordered breathing refers to a range of breathing problems that occur during sleep in children. It encompasses conditions such as mouth breathing, snoring, upper airway resistance syndrome (UARS), and obstructive sleep apnea (OSA). Now I know I just used some fancy doctor talk then, don't worry, there is a translation into mom and dad talk on the way.

Think of a hose connected to a tap. Now if you kink the hose completely, the water cannot come through. Kink it a little bit and a varying amount of water flows, depending on the degree of blockage. Well, that is sort of the same as sleep disordered breathing. I will go in to why mouth breathing is bad for the health of your child in due course, but it is the bottom rung of this spectrum. In this situation, most of the time there is a blockage to normal airflow through the nose, such that the child reverts to breathing through their mouth instead.

The next rung up is snoring. In this situation, there is still air moving in and out, but instead of it being a smooth flow of air, it is turbulent. Think of it like being at the beach, and there can be smooth water, or waves, and if there are waves, you'll hear them crashing down as they break. Well snoring is made because there is some form of obstruction. In this scenario, it is important to realize that the volume of the snoring does not directly relate to the degree of obstruction. This is easily explained by thinking about someone choking you (sorry for the confronting analogy, but bear with me). If someone is choking you a little bit, you may be able to scream and make some noise, but if they choke you a lot, then you may not be able to make much noise at all. Well, it is the same with snoring, sometimes the snoring is minimal because the obstruction is minimal, sometimes the snoring is minimal because the blockage is major.

Now about that doctor talk- Upper Airways Resistance Syndrome- what is that all about? Well Upper Airway Resistance Syndrome (UARS) is a condition characterized by partial blockage or narrowing of the upper airway during sleep. It is similar to obstructive sleep apnea (which I am coming to in a moment) but with milder symptoms. The person is however so blocked, they put extra effort than normal in to breathing to get the air in and out. So, in other words, they are struggling. This may cause the child to have frequent, partial awakenings throughout the night, leading to poor sleep quality. These awakenings are often so brief that the child or parent may not even be aware of them. As there is still airflow, there may or may not be a deprivation of oxygen that is measurably significant, at least not as much compared to obstructive sleep apnea, our next and worst type of issue in the sleep disordered breathing spectrum.

Obstructive sleep apnea is characterized by the hall mark of either a reduced amount of air going in during breathing in or no air at all, or both. The reduced airflow has a special name called a hypopnea, and the full reduction is known as an apnea. These episodes not only disturb the sleep cycles but the low oxygen supply results in a multitude of health problems, all of which will also be discussed in due course.

So what do parents need to look out for?

Again, keeping it simple, there are clues evident during the time your child is awake, but more so the main clues are when they are asleep. The latter means you need to do some spying on them once they have drifted off.

The night time clues are the obvious, such as mouth breathing, snoring, and noticing they are struggling to breathe or even stop breathing. Extra clues include sleep walking, night terrors, teeth grinding, sleep talking, restless sleep, tossing and turning through the night, sweating at night, wetting the bed beyond an age expected, starting to wet the bed again having had a period of time when it stopped, and waking up and either calling out or coming into your bedroom.

The first day time clue is waking up tired. In fact, this one thing is a major determining factor for the likelihood of your child suffering from the major list of problems I am going to be talking about very soon. The other clues that may then flow through in the day time include excessive daytime sleepiness or fatigue, morning headaches, difficulty concentrating or memory problems, struggling at school, emotional outbursts including being sad or angry, poor academic performance, and decreased physical performance during play, sport, or exercise.

That is quite a list!

But it is an important list. This is because sleep-disordered breathing is relatively common in children, with estimates suggesting that up to 20% of children may have it, and only 1 in 10 of these children are being diagnosed and treated appropriately. This condition can occur at any age, but it is more common in preschool-aged children.

So if that is the problem, what is the cause?

This is where it gets easy and then very tricky. The easy bit is most of the time it is due to tonsils and adenoids getting too big. The tricky bit is that that is not the only cause, and if a cookie cutter approach to the problem is adopted to fixing things, a good number of children will not get the correct treatment they need. The other tricky thing, is that something that caused it initially and is fixed could come back later on, or a different cause of the problem could show up down the track and lead to a relapse. I will make this easier to understand in due course.

So let's deal with the elephant in the room- large tonsils and adenoids.

The tonsils are located at the back of the throat. There is on one each side of the side wall of the throat and they can be seen by looking inside the mouth. The adenoids are located behind the nasal cavity. Despite the plural spelling of the word, there is only one adenoid. To see this, you need a special camera that passes through the nasal passages, aimed towards the back of the head. Both the tonsils and adenoids belong to a primitive and basic part of the immune system known as the MALT system. Whilst they do have an immune function, it is a very basic one and for thousands of years now the removal of these has been performed, fortunately in more recent times with the use of a general anesthetic. I will talk about surgery more later.

So why do they get too big?

Well, it was not until about 2016 that we had a reasonably good answer to that question. For a long time, we thought it was related to bacterial infections. In 2016 researchers identified viruses in enlarged tonsils and adenoids where there was a demonstrable response of the body to these viruses. So essentially the tonsils and adenoids had filtered some of these viruses but instead of the viruses being eliminated, they persisted, and the ongoing escalation of the fight against these persistent viruses led to the tonsils and adenoids getting bigger. In addition to viruses, there are some bacteria that we have identified that are implicated and also, we know that having a history of gastroesophageal reflux and exposure to cigarette smoke play a role too. If either the tonsils, or adenoids, or both get too big, they will occupy valuable space reserved for breathing. Hence why their enlargement is a real concern. But there is big difference between being the main cause of obstructed breathing and the only cause. This is why it is important to know about all of the causes, as the fix needs to be aimed towards the problem.

So what else may cause trouble breathing in children?

The next thing on the list is nasal allergies. You may know it as hay fever. Us doctors show off and call it allergic rhinitis. Fancy talk aside, the reason nasal allergies are a problem for breathing is that the allergies cause swelling of the skin lining of the inside of the nose, especially the side walls. If you have ever looked inside the nostrils of a person with allergies, you might see some red swellings; well, that's the problem right there. These red swellings get called polyps by people that do not know what they are seeing. They are not polyps. These red swellings are inflamed structures called turbinates. If the turbinates are too big, we call it enlarged turbinates (see, not all doctor talk is designed to be confusing), and to then show off we call it turbinate hypertrophy (spoke too soon, didn't I). We are going to talk about an approach to nasal allergies in due course.

Next on the list to talk about is also in the nose, and this is a scenario where the structure in the middle of the nose that separates the left and right side is crooked. This structure is known as the septum, and if it is crooked, we call it a deviated septum. My job is pretty easy, as the septum is either straight or crooked. The reason the septum becomes crooked is from some form of physical trauma. You may be surprised to learn that about 1-3% of babies have a deviated septum from the birthing process. And if you sit back and think about how many times your child has face planted, had a ball it them in the face, or other miscellaneous trauma that at the time you did not even think twice about, then you'll suddenly appreciate how your child could end up with a broken septum that becomes deviated. Again, we will talk about fixing this later on too.

Next, we have underdeveloped jaws. As there is a top and bottom jaw, any situation where one or the other does not grow properly can have an impact on the airway. Let me explain how. Starting with the top jaw, it can be either too narrow or not grow forwards adequately (or both). If it is narrow, the issue there is that the nose is based upon the upper jaw; so, a narrow jaw means a narrow nose. Furthermore, the upper jaw serves as a curtain rod for the side walls of the throat; so, a narrow upper jaw means the side walls of the throat are closer to each other, again reducing the space available. The other issue is caused if it does not grow forwards. This is because behind the nose there is a little space, and if the upper jaw is sitting back from where it should be, it makes this space smaller. Any of these scenarios leads to a reduction in the space for breathing through.

So how about the lower jaw? Well, if it does not grow outwards enough, then the tongue gets squished, and this forces it upwards, which means it pushes it up into the airway space. And if the lower jaw sits back, it pushes the tongue backwards in to the airway. So, the development of the jaws is really important, and given 80-90% of this happens from ages 8-12, we need to get in early and guide jaws in the right direction. And yes, I will talk more about this later too.

The other growing concern, literally, is obesity. Being overweight causes a range of issues in terms of health, and one of them is it makes breathing slightly more difficult to do. There are several reasons for this but 3 simple reasons are the following:

1. The extra weight around the tummy is something that the diaphragm (which is the main breathing muscle) has to push against to open up the lungs, so that means the lungs may not open up fully
2. The extra soft tissue around the neck squashes in the airway
3. The tongue tends to get fat build up in it, making it bigger.

The other common health condition that contributes to sleep disordered breathing being worse is having asthma. The links are a bit hard to explain, so I won't. Suffice to say though that part of the link is that having nasal allergies increases the chances of having asthma, so that's part of the story. The other thing to note is that it is not just that asthma can make sleep disordered breathing worse, but sleep disordered breathing can make asthma worse. So it is quite the vicious circle.

The icing on the cake to causes of sleep disordered breathing are rare things such as certain abnormalities of jaw growth that are part of a major syndrome, certain genetic diseases, and certain conditions that affect the brain, nerves, or muscles of the body. These are rather obvious in their initial presentation and such children affected by them will already be under the watchful care of a team of specialists, so for simplicity again, I will not go into the details further here.

So far, I have explained what sleep disordered breathing is, and how it can come about. The next step is to highlight what problems sleep disordered breathing may cause to a developing child. Now I will be honest, the next section may be confronting for some parents and comforting for others as they learn about what their child is struggling. So rather than be intimidated by what is coming next, use the next chapter as a means of empowering your resolve to help your child be free of obstructed breathing.

5. The consequences of sleep disordered breathing

Untreated sleep-disordered breathing can have significant consequences for a child's health and development. It can lead to chronic sleep deprivation, impaired cognitive function, behavioral problems, cardiovascular issues, growth disturbances, and decreased quality of life. These are all potentially avoidable, and the best outcomes with any condition are early diagnosis and early treatment. So let's get the journey of discovery underway, starting with the most precious thing your child will have for their whole life, their brain.

Given the brain does so many things, this is going to be quite a list, however, as much as I want to make things simple, I think this particular area of concern warrants me also being thorough as the reality is that sleep disordered breathing can have potential effects on a child's brain due to disrupted sleep patterns and intermittent oxygen deprivation.

In no particular order, let's start with how sleep-disordered breathing can have an impact a child's learning. First up, their cognitive function. Disrupted sleep patterns, frequent awakenings, and decreased oxygen levels during sleep can lead to difficulties with attention, concentration, memory, and problem-solving. The interrupted sleep and reduced oxygen levels can impair the consolidation and processing of information during sleep, which is crucial for memory and learning. Children with untreated SDB may have difficulties acquiring and retaining new knowledge, impacting their academic progress. The net effect of this is that it can show up in school aged children with their academic performance suffering. So, if you start to get feedback from the teacher that your child is struggling to concentrate in class, having difficulty staying engaged during lessons, and experiencing challenges with completing assignments or exams, then pause for a moment and ask yourself when was the last time you checked on their breathing and sleep.

The other clue that a brain that is struggling to function properly can be in the development of behavioral Issues. These themselves can also impact on learning. Children may exhibit symptoms such as hyperactivity, impulsivity, inattentiveness, restlessness, an inability to sit still, or irritability. This can manifest as constant fidgeting, squirming, or difficulty staying focused on tasks. You might be surprised to learn that research estimates 25-50% of children diagnosed as having ADHD may actually just need to get better breathing and sleep, because the symptom overlap between ADHD and a child with sleep disordered breathing is very high.

Next on the list we have something called executive function. These are specific life skills such as planning, organizing, and self-regulation. These can be compromised in children with sleep-disordered breathing. These functions are important for goal-directed behavior, problem-solving, and academic success. When sleep is disrupted, children may struggle with these skills, impacting their ability to manage their time, prioritize tasks, and meet academic expectations.

By the way, I am emphasizing the school and learning each step of the way for a reason. School attendance and engagement is very important as missed learning opportunities can hinder their overall educational progress and this has a lifelong impact on their lives, careers, and relationships. I cannot emphasize enough the importance of early detection and appropriate management of sleep disordered breathing to minimizing the impact of this condition on a child's learning abilities.

Although the above is pretty significant, let me expand even further. Sleep disordered breathing can contribute to mood swings and increased sensitivity to stressors. Such children may become easily frustrated, have emotional outbursts, or display moodiness. The disrupted sleep and poor quality of rest can impact their emotional regulation and make it more challenging for them to cope with daily challenges. So that phrase "terrible twos"; well, I am certain a lot of those children have an airway issue but are fobbed off as being two years old.

Then we have issues with impulsivity. Children with sleep disordered breathing may act on their immediate desires without considering the consequences, leading to challenges in social interactions, impulsively blurting out answers in class, or difficulty waiting their turn. A flow on effect of all of the above can be aggression and defiant behaviors. Just pause for a moment and think of what you are like the next day after a bad night's sleep. Why should it be any different for children? Actually, it is different- it is worse in children. Their brains need consistent sleep every night. And a child with sleep disordered breathing is not having just one bad night; it is pretty much every night.

Now if this is not sounding bad enough, let me seal the deal with the following statement- children with sleep disordered breathing are more likely to suffer from anxiety and depression, plus a range of other mental health disorders. Sorry. Not sorry.

To be a ray of sunshine among these dark clouds, it is important to note that the impact of sleep disordered breathing on a child's brain can vary based on the severity and duration of the condition, as well as individual factors. Hence, early identification, diagnosis, and appropriate treatment can help reduce the potential effects on a child's brain and overall development.

OK. Now let's move on to something else. The cardiovascular system. That is a fancy way of saying heart and blood vessels. And I wish what I am about to say is not as scary as the brain stuff. And it probably isn't. But it is a very close second.

Sleep-disordered breathing can have several effects on a child's heart due to the recurrent disruptions in breathing and oxygen levels during sleep. One thing that happens in children (and adults by the way) during an episode of obstructed breathing is that there is a response where the body responds by releasing adrenaline and also activates part of the nervous system called the sympathetic nervous system. This system is our body stress response- you might have heard of it and heard it called the "fight or flight" response. This activation and adrenaline release can cause an increase in blood pressure. Frequent episodes of increased blood pressure during sleep can lead to sustained high blood pressure levels, known as hypertension. Yes, that is right, children can end up with high blood pressure. Furthermore, having sleep disordered breathing a child increases the subsequent risk of having high blood pressure as an adult.

Now high blood pressure is bad for the heart. As is low oxygen levels in the blood. In each case, they put a strain on the heart. This strain is due to the increased workload required to maintain oxygen supply to the body to try compensate for the interrupted breathing plus in the case of high blood pressure, forcing the blood to flow when it is relatively resistant to do so. Over time, this strain can contribute to changes in the heart's structure and function, such as the heart getting bigger and also less efficient.

Add to this, children with untreated sleep disordered breathing have an increased risk of developing narrowing and hardening of the arteries, known as atherosclerosis, developing abnormal heart rhythms, known as arrhythmias, and they may struggle so much that their hearts start to fatigue and they develop heart failure.

The other notable area of cardiovascular disease is having a stroke. And yes, children can have strokes. And yes, having sleep disordered breathing is associated with an increased risk of having certain types of strokes as a child. Fortunately, this is very rare. So I won't dwell on it. I think enough said already actually.

Once again, it is important to note that the impact of sleep disordered breathing on a child's cardiovascular system can vary based on the severity and duration of the condition, as well as individual factors. Early identification, diagnosis, and appropriate treatment is essential.

Now let's look in another part of the body, the gut. This may seem like a strange place to consider, but in the body, everything is connected. I am going to talk about something called the gut microbiome. This is again fancy talk for bacteria that live inside of us. Most people will be aware this is the case, and if not, have fun looking it up- it is quite fascinating. It is important to highlight that the relationship between sleep-disordered breathing and the gut microbiome in children is an area of emerging research. The exact mechanisms and effects are still being investigated, but it is interesting, so I want to talk about it.

If there is an imbalance or disruption in the composition and diversity of the gut microbiome, we call this dysbiosis. Some research suggests that children with untreated sleep disordered breathing may have alterations in their gut microbiome, characterized by changes in the relative abundance and diversity of certain bacterial species. Dysbiosis can potentially affect the overall health and function of the gastrointestinal system, and maybe even the whole body itself.

One mechanism by which we think this change in the gut microbiome is brought about is by a reaction called inflammation. I haven't told you this yet, but long standing and repeated drops in the oxygen level and sleep fragmentation, can trigger widespread inflammation in the body. This inflammation is known to impact the gut microbiome and, hence, can potentially contribute to dysbiosis. To make things worse, and this is why dysbiosis is potentially very serious, dysbiosis and inflammation may then interact to influence metabolic processes in the body, such as causing insulin resistance, which elevates blood sugar levels, which may then lead to obesity. Now don't forget I mention obesity makes sleep disordered breathing worse; so, this is really a perfect storm.

The icing on the cake for this dysbiosis is that we are coming to learn there is a communication from the gut directly to the brain. This is being referred to as the Gut-Brain Axis. The significance of this communication is that disruptions in the gut microbiome, can potentially impact brain function and behavior. Given this is already something that is compromised for other reasons, the issues I am talking about are only getting worse.

But let's not get ahead of ourselves. It is important to note that further research is needed to fully understand the complex interactions I have outlined. So be alarmed but not afraid.

Still in the gut but now focusing on a specific mineral, I am going to talk about iron. Now iron is very important for our body because it is a key ingredient in the protein in our red blood cells that carries the oxygen around our bodies. If the iron is low, this could result in a reduced ability of the blood to transport iron around as the body cannot make enough of the protein that iron is an ingredient for. Combine this reduced oxygen transport ability with reduced oxygen in the first place, and you can probably see why low iron is not going to be a good thing if you also have sleep disordered breathing. As an aside, iron is also an important element used by the brain for communicating messages within itself. So yeah, also not a good thing. So, if I am talking about low iron, obviously it is for a reason. Guess what percentage of children with sleep disordered breathing have low iron. It is about 20%. That is not insignificant. So let's go chat about iron.

If the iron is low, we call this an iron deficiency. There are several reasons why children with sleep disordered breathing may end up with low iron.

The first is they may not be getting enough in their diet. Not so much by choices at home about whether they are fed meat or not, but more so that children with sleep disordered breathing have trouble chewing and swallowing meat. The struggle with chewing because firstly they may need to breathe through their mouths, so in terms of surviving they favor soft mushy foods as these are easier to clear quickly and get the next breath in. Also, children with sleep disordered breathing tend to have reduced activity and strength of the muscles that close the jaws, making chewing harder. And finally, if they have large tonsils at the back of their throat, then pushing meat past them is too difficult. Such children are in survival mode. The have learned that meat is too hard and resist it.

As if that is not enough, even if they do eat meat, the next challenge is they need a gut that works properly to absorb the iron. I highlighted how these children may have a dysbiosis of their microbiome, and this in itself may affect iron absorption. But there is more. The repeated bouts of low oxygen may lead to the release of a substance known as hepcidin. Elevated levels of hepcidin can interfere with iron absorption too. And to seal the deal, let's go back to those nasal allergies. Having a nasal allergy means you have inflammation in your body, so even without there necessarily also being an associated airway issue, nasal allergies and the inflammation associated with this can lead to low iron. Oh, and did I mention that low iron makes allergies worse? No? Well, I just did.

With all of this in mind, it seems fitting now to round off this discussion with mouth breathing. Please be aware that this is not normal. It is almost always a sign of a restriction to nasal airflow. So, it is a symptom rather than a diagnosis. However, mouth breathing, for whatever cause has some very notable effects. Let's dive in.

Chronic mouth breathing can impact the development of a child's dental and facial structures. Breathing through the mouth can lead to an open bite, where the front top and bottom teeth do not touch each other, crowded or misaligned teeth, a narrow upper jaw (which if you recall can itself lead to breathing issues through the nose), and changes in the shape and overall position of the jaws. These effects can contribute to orthodontic issues and may require intervention such as braces or orthodontic appliances. So if you are worried about such a thing happening, make sure your child is not a mouth breather.

These are not the only dental issues though. Mouth breathers are at increased of a buildup of plaque on their teeth, tooth decay, gum disease, and bad breath. They are also more likely to grind their teeth, wearing down the teeth, sometimes all the way to the nerve. As an aside low iron can also cause teeth grinding, as can having nasal allergies. You are probably seeing that these children with sleep disordered breathing don't stand much of a chance to escape its grip.

Mouth breathing can also affect a child's speech and language development. It can lead to alterations in tongue and lip movements, which may impact pronunciation and the ability to form certain speech sounds correctly. This can result in speech disorders or difficulties with clear communication. This can then lead to anxiety, poor school performance and social isolation. Once again, this is a monster that feeds on itself when it comes to affecting the child involved.

I hope you may recall that I talked about children with sleep disordered breathing sometimes having jaw muscles that do not work properly. Well, chronic mouth breathing can lead to imbalances in the facial muscles and reduced function of the muscles involved in proper nasal breathing. This can perpetuate the habit of mouth breathing and make it more challenging to transition to nasal breathing. Once again, we are going around in circles.

Now when it comes to mouth breathing, you may be surprised that I bring up the topic of tongue tie. A tongue tie describes the clinical scenario where the attachment of the undersurface of the tongue to the bottom of the mouth is too tight. Interestingly this may be a factor in some children when it comes to mouth breathing. It is not a major player in the game, but it does seem that tongue tie can contribute to or be associated with mouth breathing in some cases. The tongue plays a crucial role in maintaining proper oral posture, including resting against the palate and helping to support the upper jaw and dental arch development. When the tongue is restricted by a tongue tie, it may not rest in the correct position, leading to an open-mouth posture and mouth breathing. It's important to note that not all individuals with tongue tie will experience mouth breathing, and most cases of mouth breathing are not related to tongue tie. So I am happy to mention it, but I will do so with emphasis on keeping things in perspective. And just by the by, getting a tongue tie fixed does not offer any protection against potential tonsil and adenoid enlargement later on in life, just in case you ever get told that.

By now, I am hoping you are understanding what sleep disordered breathing is, and what problems it can cause. So the purpose here is to motivate you to check on your child and get them assessed if you suspect they may have sleep disordered breathing. In the next section, I will share what health care providers you may cross paths with and explain what their role is in terms of the assessments they may offer.

6. The importance of a comprehensive evaluation

I would expect that by now it is clear that with so many possible things going on, the desire to get things assessed is now confused by where to start. And again, I am going to make this simple- start with an ENT surgeon that focusses on the assessment and management of sleep disordered breathing. Then get a perspective from a dentist that is aware that potential abnormal jaw growth issues contribute to sleep disordered breathing. If you do these two things, you will have covered more than 90% of the worrying causes of upper airway obstruction. A clinical diagnosis typically involves a process of taking a thorough evaluation of the child's medical history, physical examination, and, if necessary, there may be some investigations called for. I will break these all down into what each person is looking for. That way you can have a list of answers ready before you even seen the first person. Also, note that I am dividing things up a little bit arbitrarily; there is no reason, for example that you may get a question from an ENT about something on the list of what to expect from a dentist.

When it comes to a clinical history, the ENT will want to know about the observed breathing issue (and hint, take a video so you can show them), how long it has been going on for, if there are episodes of stopping breathing, sleep walking, sleep talking, night terrors, teeth grinding, sweating at night, persisting or relapse of bed wetting, general energy level first thing in the morning, morning headaches, educational issues, concentration issues, behavioral issues, energy levels with physical activity, if there are any suggestions of hay fever, asthma, prematurity, or reflux, and general health issues of any other kind in the background. They will also want to know the specific ENT issues such as a history of ear infections, tonsillitis, nasal trauma, and any previous ENT surgery. The ENT should then examine the ear, nose, and throat, and this may also require the use of a special camera into the nose to get a good look at everything. Investigation wise, they may request a blood test to assess the iron levels, and they may also organize a blood test for nasal allergies. If there is uncertainty, they may advise seeing an allergy doctor to double check on any allergies in the background. Some ENT doctors are still using an X-ray to look at the adenoids; I don't. If your ENT does, just be mindful that it is a radiation dose and that there are the camera systems I mentioned which are actually a lot more accurate for assessing the adenoids. And lastly, they may or may not organize a measurement of the breathing during sleep called a sleep study. Sleep studies in children are unfortunately unreliable for several reasons, the main one being when it comes to sleep disordered breathing, they are geared to diagnosing obstructive sleep apnea and not the other types of sleep disordered breathing; so a normal sleep study does not mean normal breathing. The other reasons they are unreliable at times is that the need to be done over several nights rather than just one, as sleep varies from night to night, they are uncomfortable and can disrupt sleep, creating confusion as to why the child may not be sleeping well, and some children just pull them off and that is the end of that.

In an ideal world, I would hope that the ENT would make some form of assessment of the jaw development. In the real world, just go and see a dentist anyways. At the dental review they will want to know about the use of a dummy (pacifier is its name elsewhere in the world), breastfeeding history, history of dental trauma, reflux history, presence of mouth breathing, fluoride use, teeth brushing routine, general diet, teeth grinding, and general dental history. They will look at the teeth and jaws and make an appraisal of dental health and well-being. It is likely they will advocate x-rays and, in the mainstay, this may be simple 2D images but there is rapid progress towards taking 3D scans which have a comparable dose of radiation and as a bonus can provide images really useful for the ENT to look at as well.

Although I have focused on the ENT and dental team as the main players in the game, please also note that there are a large range of people that could form the team for your child. This includes a sleep specialist, speech and language therapist, myofunctional therapist, occupational therapist, psychologist, audiologist, allergist, dietitian, physical therapist and if I missed anyone, drop me a line and I'll add it to the list. I would encourage you to refer to your collection of health care professionals as you dream team (groan!).

So I guess this means we need to get on and actually fix this problem. Good idea.

7. Treatment Options

Call me biased, but the mainstay of fixing sleep disordered breathing in children is surgery, specifically tonsil and adenoid removal. But I made it clear early on this is not the be all and end all. What I am going to do is walk you through 4 ENT operations, allergy management, maxillary expansion and oral appliances, and myofunctional therapy, and something called CPAP. That covers the big picture and I will try and give you a suggested sequence of how to do this along the way, in terms of what gets fixed and when.

The four operations I am going to talk about are tonsillectomy, adenoidectomy, turbinate reduction, and septoplasty, in that order. It is important to emphasize a child may need none, one, or a combination of these. It is important that precise treatments are delivered to address precise issues as the appropriate treatment for pediatric sleep disordered breathing depends on its underlying cause and severity.

When it comes to tonsillectomy, parents should be aware that it is one of the most common surgical procedures performed in children and that the main reason it is done is to relieve obstruction, and not to stop attacks of tonsillitis (though that is the second most common reason for doing the procedure). A tonsillectomy is performed under general anesthesia. There are many different ways of removing the tonsils and the best method is the one your surgeon has found delivers the safest results. I have to emphasize that experience really does matter.

Since this and other operations I am going to talk about involve a general anesthetic, I am going to take a little detour and walk you through what to expect when it comes to your child having this medication; be mindful that each place may do it slightly different, this is just big picture in terms of the description. So things start before you even arrive as you will be advised in a few days prior to the procedure about your admission and fasting times.

When it comes to fasting times, I cannot highlight enough how these are totally not negotiable. There are serious dangers to having an anesthetic if the fasting procedure has not been followed diligently. You will be given 2 fasting time points- one will be food, and the other is clear liquids. Clear liquids means when it is in a glass, you can see through it. Anything else is food- this includes smoothies, milk, and obviously food. Do not mix this up, otherwise you will turn up and be made to wait. This also means you need to make sure your child does not have access to any food whatsoever in the fasting window. Sometimes that means making sure you wake up before they do and getting them out of the house away from temptation and to save you the angst of finding them in the fridge when you've turned your back for a minute. I would also advocate that you join them in the fasting journey; it is a bit mean from a child's perspective that you are eating when they are not allowed to and absolutely under no circumstances are you to eat or drink anything when you get to the hospital and you are in the waiting area with your child and probably other patients fasting and waiting for their turn for surgery.

As part of this journey, you may want to try and explain to your child what is going to happen. Let me help you out here, and without trying to sound condescending in the process; unless a child has been through this process of going to theatre in the past, most of them will have no idea what it is all about. Under no circumstances tell them "It will be scary, but you will be OK". We do not need to tell a child it will be scary. They are a blank canvas and telling them it will be scary does not make our job easier. Just let them know they are going on an adventure and everyone will just have to see what happens on the day as it is a bit of a surprise. If you are feeling anxious about it, please try and put on a brave face- children are very good at sensing fear and if they see you are worried, they will start to worry too.

In terms of what to pack and wear to hospital, I have simple suggestions. No jewelry of any kind as you will need to take it all off anyway. Do not wear your best clothes. Onesies are not great as we need to get access to the child's arm, chest, and tummy and these make doing so very difficult.

Bring one toy and make sure you know it is your responsibility to safeguard it once they are under the anesthetic, so just in case, don't bring their absolute favorite. Bring a spare pair of clothes, just in case your child wets themselves when they are asleep. If they have certain food requirements or preferences, bring those along for after the procedure too. If they are on any medications, bring those in, just in case, and in such circumstances clarify with the anesthetist about whether it is safe to continue using medications up to and including the day of surgery, or whether anything needs to be stopped or the dose adjusted. And lastly, bring something you can distract them with whilst you're waiting. I can guarantee you that there is no specific time that you absolutely will go in to theatre. We all make estimates and that is an educated guess. It is not an absolute and chances are you will be sitting around waiting a while.

Once you have arrived, you will finalize paperwork and then be asked to take your seat and wait your turn- well I did just warn you, didn't I? Please note that there are no cameras, phones, or filming in the surgery theatre, so get all of your pictures sorted before that moment. At some stage you will meet the doctor that administers the anesthetic, and all being OK, you will be shortly taken into the operating theatre. Here is where the magic happens and it is super important that you let the professionals do their job. Now some places will let you come in with your child, and others don't. Either way I will cover what happens inside, just to cover the scenario that a place lets you come in. In doing so let me preempt a few things. Firstly, if you are anxious and panicked then please do not come in. It will only make things harder for us, not easier; as much as you may feel being there for you child is important, the research shows no difference in how a child transitions through theatre, and recovery, and their take home feeling about the experience whether you are there or not as they go off to sleep. I am just saying this because you need to understand this is a critical moment of care of your child and we really need a clear pathway forward to do this with absolute safety in mind.

OK, so we are in theatre and your child is on the bed. Next comes the mask. This initially is just oxygen, a standard step before any general anesthetic. Next, we have the going off to sleep, and there are 2 ways this may be done. Most commonly in children it is with gas, and the alternative is via medication through a tube inserted into one of their veins; as most children are not great with needles, and a needle is part of the process to insert this tube, this is why we tend to use gas first, get them to sleep, and then put the needle in without them knowing. If it is the needle, it is really quick- like less than 30 seconds quick. Gas takes a bit longer, and as a result there is a wind down period where different part of the brain shut off. The first part of the brain to shut off is the awareness part. So even though they still have their eyes open and are looking around, they have no recollection once their awareness is switched off. During this period they may even move around, call out, and look to be in a state of panic; this is just a sign of their brain being confused, and it is not nice to see but it is normal; often for their own safety we will have a few of us hold the child down to prevent them from accidentally falling off the bed as they wriggle. They may also tray and pull the mask off, and again we will gently restrain them from doing so as we do not want to end up in a situation where we cannot be providing them with additional oxygen. Then very shortly after the wriggle stage, they pass out. At that point we take over and you will be asked to leave. Please do so promptly as we have things that we need to do quickly and again, it is not a thing we let parent see because by about now that is about as much trauma parents can take and the tears are often starting to flow. Rest assured they are in good hands and they are the best hands if they are not distracted. The next time you see your child will be in recovery.

So let's jump to the recovery room. The waking up process is like the going to sleep process- it can be quite tumultuous. As a result, you will not be there when you child is starting to wake up. And they will not know if you are there or not due to the medications they have had. In fact, they will not remember much of the first few hours when they are waking up and recovering. So you being there is not important to them, in terms of making a difference to how they wake up. Now about that waking up bit. In about 20% of children, they wake up in a transition zone as to which parts of their brains have recovered from the anesthetic, and it is random as to the order different bits switch on. As a result, there is a potential for something called "emergence delirium", and like I said it happens about 20% of the time. If this happens, your child will be inconsolable, panicked, disorientated, and may show off their swear word vocabulary that you never knew they had, and call you names and say they hate you. This is obviously not a fun ride for anyone but the one redeeming thing is your child will not remember any of this. So be prepared but not alarmed, it does pass should you get the short straw.

Now where was I? Oh yes, tonsillectomy....

As I was saying, tonsillectomy is generally considered safe, but like any operation, it is not without risks. The one complication that we face more than any other is bleeding in the 2-week recovery period after this surgery. Now a little bit of bleed is normal. In 1-4% of cases a little bit becomes a lot, and a lot means a trip back to hospital, possibly needing medication, or surgery again, and rarely a blood transfusion. It is an unfortunate reality that this can happen, but it is better to be forewarned to be forearmed. I always advise my patients having this operation are no more than one hour away from a major hospital service able to manage such an emergency for the whole of those two weeks after the operation.

During those 2 weeks, pain and discomfort are common after a tonsillectomy, and apart from a sore throat, ear pain and difficulty swallowing are not uncommon. They get ear pain because the nerve to the tonsils also connects in to the ear, and the brain gets mixed up as to where the pain is coming from, and confuses it as coming from the ears. As the child recovers, it is typical for the pain to escalate at approximately day 4-6 after surgery, and when it does, for this to last 2-3 days, and then things start to settle. It is super important to administer regular pain relief. You are trying to stop the pain from happening, rather than trying to settle it down once it is there. Some children will go into being defiant, a symptom of their sleep disordered breathing, and refuse the pain relief. The only potential way around this is to administer the pain relief as a suppository formulation (that means putting it in their bottom- and it's funny how when I tell parents that, how much more determined they become to get the oral mediation in to their child). If a child refuses pain relief, there is nothing you can do. There is an easy way and a hard way through the recovery, and some children just become their own worst enemy. They will get better just the same in due course. As to the type of pain relief used, I have avoided the use of strong opiate drugs for the past 30 years. The research shows it makes no difference to overall pain scores, and actually increases the possibility of complications such as nausea, vomiting, constipation, and sadly even death. I know it sounds weird, but I would rather a child is alive.

In terms of what else to expect during the recovery, the child will be miserable, flat, and getting them to eat and drink will be a challenge. They will have bad breath and temperatures, and with all of this going on, your plan ahead of time should be to rest up at home, no visitors, no physical activity, stay out of the heat if it is hot weather, no exposure to cigarette smoke, and just let them eat and drink whatever they want with the ideal being a return to a normal diet as quick as possible. At the end of the day though, keeping up fluids is the most important, so if it is a struggle, have a small syringe available as one of the tricks it to sit with your child and set a timer so every minute you give them 1-10mls (also known as cc) every minute. In an hour you could end up giving them quite a good amount of fluid using this trick.

The last trick I have to share to get through a tonsillectomy is to elevate the child as they sleep with an extra pillow or two. This reduces swelling in the throat, and this in turn reduced the pressure and pain in the surgical area. Needless to say, recovering from a tonsillectomy can be a challenging experience for a child. Providing emotional support, reassurance, and comforting activities can help ease their anxiety or discomfort during the recovery period. And ice cream. Lots of ice cream. Or ice blocks or the like if they are dairy intolerant.

I know this all sounds very dramatic but what I have done is paint the worst-case scenario for you. For most of you, this will not be the case and you will bounce through relatively unscathed. Like I said, I would rather you are forewarned, just in case you get the short straw.

So having talked about tonsillectomy, I have good news- all of the other procedures are nowhere near as bad in terms of the recovery process. So you have just read about the worst of it. Let's discuss adenoidectomy.

To remind you, the adenoids are located at the back of the nasal cavity. It is often done with tonsil surgery, and if that is the case, there is so much more going on with the tonsil recovery that you won't even notice the adenoids being an issue. Apart from removing the adenoids for airway obstruction, we also remove them if there have been issues with infection, such as sinus issues or middle ear infections. Once again this is done under general anesthesia. The approach to the adenoids is mostly via the mouth, sometimes via the nose. There are again different ways of doing the operation, and again it comes down to experience. I would highlight one important thing though, clarify with your surgeon before you book surgery with how they visualize the adenoids as part of the procedure; the reason for bringing this to your attention is that the most common way of removing the adenoids is to scrape them out, but in doing so, most people then do not look at if the adenoids have been removed entirely, rather they do it by feel, which has been shown to be less reliable than looking. There are 2 ways of looking- using a mirror or using a camera; either is fine, it is just important that it is done.

The recovery from an adenoidectomy alone is pretty straight forward. A mild sore throat is normal, but nothing so bad it interferes with eating or drinking. Temperatures and bad breath for a few days are also par for the course. Again, the use of simple and regular pain relief makes the recovery easier.

And that's about it. Adenoidectomy really is a low-end procedure, with some very rare risks, so rare I am going to let your specialist tell you about the ones they think are worthwhile you knowing about.

Tonsil and adenoid surgery alleviate airway obstruction, at least in the short term, in about 80% of children. There are two other ENT operations that sometimes come in to play, and both of these relate to the nose. Again, these are nothing as dramatic to tonsillectomy when it comes to the recovery process, so if they are done with tonsil surgery then the tonsils will be the more noticeable element in the recovery.

The first nasal operation I am going to talk about is surgery on the nasal turbinates, and more specifically and anatomically correct in their description, the inferior nasal turbinates. If you have forgotten what these are, then this is a perfect moment to pause and rewind back to chapter 4.

There are several types of inferior nasal turbinate surgery. The two I want to cover quickly offer short term relief, have a relapse rate, and are lesser used by me these days. The first is called turbinate cautery, where the skin lining over the turbinate is burnt by the application of heat. This initially causes swelling and a runny nose but then the tissue scars up and in turn this shrinks the turbinate. I use this in children under the age of 3-4 years of age simply because the equipment otherwise won't fit inside their nose. I am not a huge fan of it otherwise as its results are quite temporary, with relapses in 6-12 months not uncommon. The other one is a similar procedure but with a bit of cool technology called radio-frequency ablation; the details do not matter but the principal outcome of soft tissue swelling shriveling up is the same, the difference is it lasts about 2 years.

The turbinate operation I want to emphasize if called a submucous turbinate reduction. This involves the physical removal of the excess tissue build up on the turbinate, and a very small piece of supporting bone. I do not take the whole turbinate out, as it is an important part of the nose for humidifying the air we breathe, and likewise I do not take too much as doing so can lead to abnormal flow of air through the nose (like the old saying, you can have too much of a good thing), and this abnormal airflow can lead to some people feeling like their nose is still blocked.

I like this procedure for several reasons: it delivers the best airway result, it tends to last forever, and in cases where they relapse, it is usually about 5 years or so down the track. In terms of post-op recovery, it is generally not painful, and the main hassle for a week or so is the nose tends to bleed on and off, rarely somewhat impressively, but in the mainstay such bleeding is managed with medication and basic first aid measures.

This surgery, and indeed all of the operations I am discussing, generally takes a few weeks for the child and family to notice the full benefits of the procedure. During the recovery phase I find using saline sprays in the nose offer some benefits. Talking of benefits, the aim of the surgery is to improve nasal airflow. Hence, it is important to note that the procedure may not completely eliminate all nasal symptoms or address underlying causes such as allergies. I will be talking about allergy management soon enough,

The last operation I will discuss of pediatric sleep disordered breathing is septoplasty. Now there is some controversy here that is worth knowing about. The historical teaching is that performing a septoplasty on a growing child is ill advised as there is a risk of compromising facial growth and development. Everything I do is risk versus benefit. I will come to that risk again shortly but let's look at the risk of not fixing a septum in a child that has symptomatic nasal obstruction caused by this structural abnormality. That is essentially everything in chapter 5. The brain. The cardiovascular. The gut. And the potential issues of mouth breathing causing an alteration in facial growth and development. That's right, the very thing we are taught to worry about happening if we fix it is also the thing we need to worry about if we do not fix it. I have been doing septal surgery for over 15 years in children. I would rather they can breathe.

So let's walk through a septoplasty. Full anesthetic, no changes to the outside of the nose, no black eyes or bruises. The surgical incisions are all internal. Post-operative pain is minimal, sometimes a bit of bleeding but not too much if done by itself, but having said that it is most commonly done in conjunction with a turbinate reduction, so they do end up getting a blood nose after but this is the turbinates' fault. Again, there are otherwise a few rare things that can happen, as is the case with any surgery, but your surgeon will decide on what to highlight to you.

That is surgery in a nutshell. So, the next thing on the list to cover is nasal allergies, properly known as allergic rhinitis, commonly known as hay fever. This describes a situation where there is an allergic reaction that occurs when the immune system overreacts to allergens (the fancy name for what causes an allergy) in the environment. The most common allergens include grass, pollen, house dust mites, pet dander, and mold. People talk about foods but this is more a sensitivity than an allergy, so I am leaving food off the list of further discussion.

The symptoms of allergic rhinitis include nasal congestion, sneezing, runny nose, itching in the nose, throat, or eyes, watery eyes, and a postnasal drip. The trick to comprehensive management of allergic rhinitis is identifying the specific allergens that trigger these symptoms, and the definitive way to do this is by allergy testing. When it comes to such testing, there are two accepted methods- a blood test (which we call a RAST) and a skin prick test. In the first, the blood it taken and an assessment is made to see if there are immune antibodies that the body has created to attack allergens. In the second, a small scratch is made on the skin and the potential cause of the allergy is applied to that scratch to see if a local allergic reaction develops; in the latter multiple small scratches are made to ensure multiple things can be tested for. Given there are millions of things that people can be allergic to, and we have a limited number that we can actually do something about, we only test for those things that we can do something about. So sometimes we know there is allergic rhinitis but we never find the culprit.

In terms of managing allergic rhinitis, there are a few strategies. One obvious one is avoidance. Sometimes this is easier said than done. For example, there are a host of things to reduce house dust mite exposure, but you will never completely out run them. Mold is everywhere. And the suggestion that the beloved family pet is the source of illness creates some inner conflicts as to the value of the child versus the offending animal.

The next line of management is medication. By far the number one medication parents tend to reach for is antihistamines. I am sorry to advise that this is well intentioned but wrong; at least in an ideal world. The first line medication for allergic rhinitis is anti-inflammatory nasal steroid sprays. These go directly into the nose and work in the nose to tackle the problem head on. Now of course, reality and ideal are not the same, but I do at least want to just let you know what you should be trying first. Antihistamines are supposed to be a top up to these sprays to manage what we call break through symptoms. The use of a nasal saline spray can also be useful, as it helps to clean the nose out, reducing the amount of allergens sitting on the skin lining of the nose. Under no circumstances should you use a nasal decongestant in a child, except under medical advice with a strict set of instructions; these medications are addictive and overuse will lead to causing a problem in the nose that is actually quite hard to fix.

As much as medications help, they are purely band-aids in terms of calming down the symptoms. They do not fix allergies. The treatment designed to help a patient get used to their allergen such that over time they need no or minimal medication is called immunotherapy, or desensitization. You may have heard of it called "allergy shots". In the mainstay, immunotherapy is done by regular injections, however there are alternatives such as drops under the tongue or oral administered tablets. Immunotherapy is not a quick fix- it can take years, but the benefits are enormous in the long term to a very high percentage of people, and it baffles me why there are not more people bashing down the doors of allergy doctors to get their children on to it; who knows, maybe once this book is out, there will be a stampede to do just that.

As a further benefit, as asthma and allergic rhinitis often co-exist, asthma management becomes easier once immunotherapy is on board in many patients. And as having allergic rhinitis can lead to developing asthma, it is beneficial to know that immunotherapy also reduces the risk of developing asthma later on. It really is a win-win-win. Yes, there can be some rare side effects, and yes in some people it disappointingly does not work so well, but life is somewhat like that in general, namely not perfect. A doctor trained in allergy management is definitely someone I value and use very frequently to deliver optimized results to my patients.

To round off allergy management, I want to put in into context with turbinate surgery, given it is the turbinates that are the things mostly affected by nasal allergies. I see this is a two-stage process- surgery to get them breathing again, and allergy management to reduce the chances of the allergy swelling coming back. The specific order and timing of each is not so important, but getting both done is a sensible package of care.

Now it is time to move away from doctors of the body and talk about doctors of the teeth, technically known as dentists. In this specialty there are two broad points of discussion- widening the jaws, specifically the upper jaw, and the use or special oral appliances to help guide the lower jaw forwards. The latter is easy to discuss in a few words- the dentist will advise the use of the appliance they have the most experience and success with, so don't fret about what the appliance is as much as what the experience of the prescriber is. As for the former, the upper jaw is called the maxilla, and making it wider is called maxillary expansion. Let's take a look at it.

Maxillary expansion is also known as palatal expansion in some circles. The aim is to widen the upper jaw. It may be part of an overall orthodontic plan, but as I am not a dentist, I just focus on its value in proving the jaw structure. If you recall, a narrow top jaw means a narrow nose; so widen the jaw, widen the nose. The device that creates this outcome is called an expander, and again there are different ones out there. The expansion process typically takes a few weeks to several months, depending on the treatment plan. There is a time critical element to getting the jaws in the right position, as 80-90% of jaw growth is done by the ages of 8-12 years. This means maxillary expansion is most effective when performed during the growth and development phase, typically before puberty. I think the ideal age for an initial assessment of potential abnormal jaw development issues is 4-6 years of age; intervention may not necessarily occur at that stage, but I see no harm in getting some baseline observations to then see what happens over time and if things are off course and drifting more so over time, then the writing is on the wall and help can be delivered sooner rather than later; the alternative down the track is major jaw surgery, so getting in early is a better option in my mind.

As for timing relative to ENT surgery, I think it is important to let the ENT go first. Maxillary expansion seems to work better if the child is given a nasal airway that works, so having an improved airway as a foundation to build upon. Plus, they are breathing better, which is not a bad thing. It is also important to note that ENT interventions are not a substitute for dental therapies, and dental therapies are not a substitute for ENT procedures. The number of parents conflicted about which one of these to proceed with is fraught with confusing messages aimed at parents keen to have a quick fix (surgery) or to avoid an operation (dental therapies). This is not a one or the other perspective; it is do the right thing for the right problem, and if that happens to be one, or the other, or both, then that is the answer to the problem at hand.

As I often say, I am not a dentist. It is important to note that maxillary expansion may be part of a comprehensive orthodontic treatment plan. Following the expansion phase, the child may require braces or other orthodontic appliances to align the teeth and achieve optimal results. My perspective is about the jaws being in the right place- they teeth can follow after. It is the jaw structure that is important in the short and then long term for breathing. I can only share my dismay one day when I saw a before and after picture of a child in an orthodontic clinic where they child had beautifully straight teeth but narrow jaws, bags under their eyes, and their gums in the picture were inflamed from mouth breathing. So, if your child is having orthodontics for crooked teeth, use this information proactively to make sure that the treating practitioner is aware of jaw structure and the importance of breathing and if they are dismissive of this concept, please consider another opinion as getting things right the first time is the best option.

Once we get to the stage of the ENT and dental team being involved, there is another important aspect of therapy, and that is rehabilitation. This brings me to myofunctional therapy, also known as orofacial myofunctional therapy. This is a specialized treatment approach that focuses on the muscles and functions of the face, mouth, and throat. It involves exercises and techniques designed to improve orofacial muscle strength, coordination, and function. Myofunctional therapy is typically conducted by a certified orofacial myofunctional therapist or a healthcare professional with specific training in this area.

The benefits of myofunctional therapy vary, which means the goals of myofunctional therapy can vary depending on the individual's needs. One of the most important elements of myofunctional therapy is to correct improper oral habits that may contribute to oral and facial muscle dysfunction. These habits can include mouth breathing, thumb sucking, tongue thrusting (where the tongue pushes forward against or between the teeth during swallowing or at rest), and improper swallowing patterns. In the context of mouth breathing, the focus is on promoting nasal breathing. Myofunctional therapy may also be recommended as a complementary treatment to orthodontic care. By improving orofacial muscle function and eliminating detrimental habits, it can enhance the effectiveness of orthodontic treatment and help maintain treatment outcomes. Given we may well need to help a child with sleep disordered breathing on their airway and orthodontic care, this therapy is invaluable to a comprehensive approach to patient wellbeing.

Myofunctional therapy typically involves regular sessions with a trained therapist, who guides the individual through exercises and techniques tailored to their specific needs. These exercises may include tongue exercises, lip exercises, breathing exercises, and swallowing exercises. The therapy often incorporates education, behavioral modification strategies, and home exercises to reinforce progress made during therapy sessions. It is a team effort, and the parent needs to be on board to make sure the child is diligent in seeing through the course of therapy.

The time has now come to discuss one more common option for managing sleep disordered breathing and that is the use of a device known as continuous positive airway pressure (CPAP). Now none of the following is intended to disparage this therapy and to sway people in to not using it; it is intended though to highlight some issues that parents should be aware of in weighing up the use of such therapy in a growing child.

To start with, CPAP is a therapy that involves the wearing of a mask at night. This allows a machine to pump air in and to try and hold the airways open. I must emphasize that this does not fix the cause of the obstruction, it just works around it; finding and fixing the cause should be the primary step in getting things back on track. Such masks may be uncomfortable or intrusive, especially in children, plus the pumping of air into their noses and mouth can take some time to adjust too; these issues may actually then compromise sleep quality. Another potential issue with the mask is that in some children they may develop skin irritation or pressure sores due to the contact of the mask with their face. As you may also expect, the likelihood of a child taking their CPAP to sleep over at their friend's house or on a school camp is somewhat unlikely. And there is also a parental burden with these machines, as they require regular maintenance and cleaning to ensure proper functioning and hygiene.

The other balancing act with the use of CPAP in a child is the potential concern that the application of a mask that is strapped on to the face may restrict the ability of the jaws to grow forwards correctly; something that is counter-productive to what we are trying to advocate for. Now to put this into context, the extent and significance of these changes are still subject to debate, and there is no consensus in the literature. Regardless, if your child is in CPAP, they must also be under the vigilant care of a dentist that will monitor for possible adverse effects such as this. As is the case with any healthcare problem, it's important to note that the potential effects of CPAP on facial growth should be weighed against the risks associated with untreated sleep-related breathing disorders in children. The negative consequences of untreated obstructive sleep apnea, such as developmental delays, cognitive impairments, and cardiovascular issues, can outweigh the potential impact on facial growth when weighing up the options.

With all of this going on, as if this is not enough to contemplate already, there is an important element that you as a parent have to play, and that is working towards creating a good space physically and mentally for your child to get the decent sleep they need. This is going to bring us to something called sleep hygiene.

8. Strategies for parents to support their child's sleep health

Sleep hygiene is an overarching term for a host of strategies to optimize sleep quality and quantity. Essentially it is about promoting healthy sleep habits and providing an environment that facilitates good sleep. As there is quite a list of things parents can do to facilitate good sleep for their child, this is again going to be simple but thorough.

When it comes to sleep habits, a crucial element is ensuring a consistent sleep schedule. This means have a firm and regular time for going to bed and waking up. For children, this entails making sure they are getting close to 10 hours of sleep per night. The routine should be consistent throughout the week, including the weekends. If your child is needing to sleep in on the weekend to catch up on their sleep, this may well be a symptom of a sleep quality or quantity issue. The reason this routine is important is that our bodies run on their own internal body clock, and we are trying to get it to align correctly by having a stable pattern of sleep-wake cycles.

In the lead up to getting in to bed, there should be an established routine of things that act as cues to the brain that sleep is to be commenced shortly. This could include reading a book, taking a bath, or listening to calming music. The big thing to avoid is stimulating activities such as electronic devices. These provided excessive light to the brain (making it think it is not dark outside, the relevance of which I will chat about a bit more shortly) plus the stimulation of the actual activity on the screen can ramp up the brain; video games are a perfect example of a bad option prior to sleeping. The aim should be to try to avoid using electronic devices for at least an hour before bed, ideally 2 hours.

Getting regular exercise can help promote better sleep. However, exercising too close to bedtime may make it difficult to fall asleep, so, if possible, aim to get this out of the way early on, and try not to let it push out the time of going to bed to later than the established routine.

Stress and anxiety can significantly impact sleep quality. This is obviously very relevant, as I have highlighted how sleep disordered breathing can elevate the likelihood of a child developing an anxious disposition. The other concern is that the brain, in its wisdom, comes to learn that sleeping leads to an inadequate supply of oxygen if there is an airway obstruction. So it solves this by trying to avoid sleep, the very thing it actually needs. Mix this in with possible defiance in a child and you have the making for yet another perfect storm. Managing stress and anxiety involves strategies such as practicing relaxation techniques and if needs be, engaging a psychologist. A relaxing pre-sleep routine will help your child's mind unwind before bed too.

Another important lifestyle measure to facilitate good sleep is to avoid large meals and fluids before bed. A full tummy can lead to some discomfort when lying down, and fluid intake at night time may add to the propensity to have to wake and go to the toilet, disrupting the sleep pattern.

The next aspect of sleep hygiene is the bedroom itself. It is important for the room to be dark. The brain has a sensor that picks up on how much light there is, and for thousands of years used the setting of the sun as a cue to start the sleep process. Artificial lighting has corrupted this process, as has the advent of screens. This also means that those night lights you thought were a good idea, actually are not so great. The other important aspect of the room is that there should be minimal noise intruding into the bedroom. This is also stimulating, and can keep a child awake. A third element of attack is to make sure the room is not too warm. The body equates a cooling of the air with the setting of the sun, and uses the temperature drop of this as another signal to get to sleep; obviously rug up on those cold nights, but don't have the temperature beyond what is a comfortable level to sit on the edge of being cool.

The last element of the bedroom is the bed and pillows. The mattress should be comfortable and supportive. Likewise, the pillow. If your child has allergies, then for dust mites there are special coverings for the mattress and pillow, and for animals they should be excluded from the room entirely to prevent animal dander finding its way to where your child rests their head.

9. Monitoring progress and evaluating treatment effectiveness

I hope the preceding discussion gives you the information and tools you need to have a road map to getting your child to breathe and sleep well. However, there can be moments where progress that was favorable takes a turn backwards; what I am talking about here is a relapse of airway obstruction.

When I contemplate a relapse, I try and look at it exactly the same as what has already been outlined- essentially start from the beginning. To elaborate, what ENT issues were identified previously, and what was done to fix them is a good start. Is it possible, for example, that the adenoids have grown back? Then I look at whether a new ENT condition has arisen. This could be tonsils that were not big initially that have increased in size; it could be the development of nasal allergies; it could be nasal trauma that makes the septum grow crooked. Then it is the dentistry side of things- is either the top or bottom jaw not developing properly? And lastly, are there other medical factors in play, in particular the development of weight gain leading to the child being overweight or obese. Are there issues with sleep hygiene confounding things too? If anything of the above is identified, this needs to be managed as already discussed. In the cases of uncertainty, the role of a sleep study and review by a pediatric sleep specialist is valuable to make sure there are no other sleep disorders in the background.

And there we have it. With things covered, the next thing to walk you through my answers to the many questions I get asked often. The answers are much already in what I have written, but it is nice to have a reminder and context to things.

10. Common Concerns and FAQs

What are the signs and symptoms of sleep-disordered breathing in children?

The most important things to look for at night are mouth breathing, snoring, and episodes of choking where the breathing stops. Tired in the morning is a red flag. Other signs may be a change in behavior, education troubles, reduced exercise capacity, emotional outbursts, and concentration lapses.

How is sleep-disordered breathing diagnosed in children?

A thorough history and examination are the cornerstone of diagnosis. A video of the child sleeping is very useful too. Certain tests may also be required, with a sleep study one worth considering, especially if there is uncertainty as to the diagnosis.

What are the potential causes or risk factors for sleep-disordered breathing in children?

The ENT causes are mostly the tonsils and adenoids, then the turbinates and nasal septum. Dental issues are jaws that do not grow forwards or outwards enough. Being overweight does not help, and conditions like asthma and nasal allergies and reflux tend to make things worse.

What are the potential consequences or complications of untreated sleep-disordered breathing in children?

Every body system and organ suffer some form of consequence to having sleep disordered breathing. The main areas featured in this book are the brain, cardiovascular system, and the gut.

Is my child's snoring normal, or could it be a sign of a sleep disorder?

Snoring when tired or unwell is not unusual. It is snoring that is evident on a regular basis without these two circumstances prevailing that should raise the concern of the parent and prompt close observation every night for 1-2 weeks, about 10-15 minutes per night, to see if it is indeed persisting.

What treatment options are available for sleep-disordered breathing in children?

It is important to address the cause. It may involve surgery, dental interventions, allergy management, medications, myofunctional therapy, weight loss strategies, and CPAP.

How effective are the different treatment options, such as CPAP, adenotonsillectomy, or orthodontic interventions?

These are all very effective treatments, but only if utilized appropriately. None are interchangeable for the other and comprehensive multidisciplinary care is more likely than any one modality to comprehensively manage this disease.

Are there any lifestyle changes or strategies that can help improve my child's sleep-disordered breathing?

Maintaining a healthy weight through diet and exercise is important. Environmental measures to control allergies is beneficial. Sleep hygiene is very important, and this involves having set routines and a bedroom environment conducive to getting good sleep.

Will my child outgrow sleep-disordered breathing, or is it likely to persist into adulthood?

We are understanding more and more that having this disease in early childhood increases the future likelihood of developing issues of a similar nature as an adult. So they grow into the problem more than outgrow it. A proactive approach early on is likely to deliver they best chances of a future life free of breathing and sleep issues.

Are there any long-term effects on my child's growth, development, or overall health due to sleep-disordered breathing?

Yes. Children with sleep disordered breathing generally tend to have a reduced amount of physical growth, tend to have learning delays, and are at increased risk of developing chronic health issues later on, such as high blood pressure for example.

What resources or support groups are available for parents of children with sleep-disordered breathing?

This book! I also have written 2 other books; one is called "Snored to Death" and it goes into a lot more detail than what is presented here and it also discussed the adult version of this disease; the other is called "Don't ignore the snore" and it details the health consequences in far more detail than here. Both are available through Amazon.

Is this a problem at any age?

Yes, it is; in fact, the younger the child when problems start, the worse their outcomes tend to be. So never think they are too young. They are not too young to get it fixed either.

What about mouth taping?

This is generally not recommended for young children or those who are unable to understand and follow instructions. Children need to have the cognitive ability to remove the tape if they experience any discomfort or difficulty breathing during the night. Never do this until an ENT has assessed the nasal airway, as often mouth breathing is a symptom of some form of obstruction.

I heard that taking the tonsils out leads to more infections later on because it is part of the immune system.

This is a myth perpetuated through time. There is one paper that suggested maybe an extra cold or 2 when older, but trade that against the effects on the brain and heart if left untreated, the balance is strongly in favor of getting oxygen in to the child.

I also heard there may be a link to developing autoimmune diseases if the tonsils are removed.

The link between tonsillectomy (surgical removal of the tonsils) and autoimmune diseases is a topic of ongoing research and debate. While there have been some observations suggesting a potential association, the relationship is complex and not fully understood. Some studies have suggested that tonsillectomy may affect the balance of the immune system, leading to alterations in immune responses and potentially increasing the risk of developing autoimmune diseases. However, the exact mechanisms by which tonsillectomy could influence autoimmune disease development are not well-established. It's important to note that tonsillectomy is often performed due to recurrent tonsillitis or sleep-disordered breathing. These underlying conditions themselves have been linked to various health issues, including autoimmune diseases. Therefore, it is challenging to determine whether the increased risk observed in some studies is directly due to tonsillectomy or related to the underlying conditions that necessitated the surgery. What we need to do is look at what happens to a group of children that had sleep disordered breathing that was not treated; it is speculative but if there underlying issue is the inflammation, then we might actually see a decreased rate of autoimmune disease in those treated versus untreated. In the meantime, again the benefits are overwhelming.

I am still not sure. I heard the tonsils and adenoids get smaller over time by themselves.

This is another bit of misinformation. It stems from some research done about 100 years ago where a body organ that is part of the immune system was studied- this organ is called the thymus. And it is true to say it gets smaller over time. This finding was then applied to the tonsils and adenoids. In fact, the tonsils and adenoids were never studied but that was the conclusion all the same. Despite this, normal and healthy tonsils and more so adenoids do indeed seem to get smaller over time; be mindful though that normal and healthy tonsils and adenoids are not the ones causing these breathing problems. Lastly, any such reduction in size tends to be slow; children with an obstructed airway do not have the luxury of time.

You freaked me out about the brain changes. Are they permanent?

The research shows two things- the earlier in life that an airway obstruction starts, and the longer it goes for, the worse the outcomes seem to be. There are documented improvements in brain function across all age groups, including adults. The best way to allay your concerns about this is to get your child seen and assessed and managed proactively. Try not to let your anxieties compromise the benefits that treating this problem can deliver.

I think I have this problem too. What should I do?

First and foremost, see an ENT- get the airway assessed. Be mindful that upper airway obstruction is not managed by all ENTs the same way. This is not unusual; find the provider most aligned to managing this condition would be my advice, even if it means travelling.

They had surgery but are still mouth breathing.

First up, give it 3 months for things to reset. Secondly, was everything fixed the way it should have been. For example, were the adenoids visualized as part of the removal process? Was the nose assessed for allergies or a deviated septum? Has there been a new problem for example has your child hit their nose during the recovery process? Were the jaws assessed to ensure they were developing correctly? And has myofunctional therapy for rehabilitation been advocated to get the child accustomed to breathing through their nose? Failing all of that, see the ENT again or get a second opinion from a different ENT to have things reassessed.

11. Conclusion and Hope for the Future

Thank you for investing your time and money in learning about sleep disordered breathing. I have done my best to give you a broad range of strategies to put in to motion to help your child. My next request to become an advocate for this condition. I want you to help me promote awareness and support for children with sleep-disordered breathing. This could be by way of sharing this information with other parents. If you are a teacher, health care professional, or in fact just anyone that works with children in some way, make the parents of children aware that sleep is important. And so is breathing.

The tonsil song

In the back of your throat, two guardians reside,

Tonsils, they're there, side by side.

But when troubles arise, it's time to take action,

A tonsillectomy, a surgical solution.

Preparation begins, a visit to the doc,

Explaining the procedure, a detailed talk.

Surgery day arrives, a mix of nerves and hope,

With skilled hands and care, they'll help you cope.

A little bit of rest, as you recover in bed,

Soothing ice cream, popsicles, and meds.

Some discomfort, but it will soon fade away,

As your throat heals, you'll be up and on your way.

No more recurrent infections, no more sleepless nights,

Breathing freely, pure delights.

With those tonsils gone, you'll feel the change,

A healthier path, a brand-new range.

Tonsillectomy, a journey to heal,

Removing those tonsils, a new chapter we'll reveal.

Singing goodbye to the pain, the discomfort, and strife,

Tonsillectomy, a step towards a better life.

So let us sing this song, a celebration so bright,

To those who've gone through the tonsillectomy fight.

Embrace the healing, the joy it brings,

Tonsillectomy, a dawn of new beginnings

Somebody's snoring

A child is sound asleep, but something's not quite right,

A snoring sound is heard, throughout the night.

It may seem innocent, but it's worth a close check,

As snoring in children, can lead to sleep wreck.

Snoring child, a sound that's not quite mild,

It may signal a problem, that needs to be filed.

Sleep apnea, or mouth breathing,

A closer examination, will find the cause of the heaving.

A visit to the doctor, a sleep study is in sight,

Measuring the breathing, throughout the night.

A diagnosis is made, a treatment plan in tow,

Ensuring the child, can breathe easy and grow.

A snoring child, a wake-up call to heed,

Addressing the issue, can help them succeed.

A better night's sleep, and a healthier life,

Is worth the effort, to end the strife.

With treatment in place, the snoring fades away,

A peaceful night's sleep, is here to stay.

No more restless nights, for child and parent alike,

A snoring child, now a thing of the past, a striking respite.

So please listen closely, to the sounds of the night,

A snoring child, a signal that all is not right.

A simple checkup, can bring about a change,

A healthier child, a life that's rearranged.

Made in United States
Troutdale, OR
09/05/2024

22595212R10037